I0766685

Why is Everyone Whispering around Me?

My Love for You goes beyond My Dementia Diagnosis

James "JEB" Butler

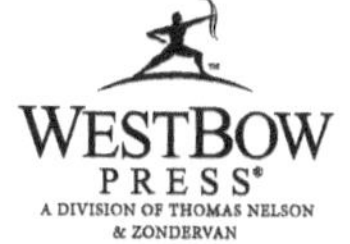

WESTBOW
PRESS®
A DIVISION OF THOMAS NELSON
& ZONDERVAN

WestBow Press books may be ordered through booksellers or by contacting:

WestBow Press
A Division of Thomas Nelson & Zondervan
1663 Liberty Drive
Bloomington, IN 47403
www.westbowpress.com
1 (866) 928-1240

Because of the dynamic nature of the Internet, any web addresses or
links contained in this book may have changed since publication and
may no longer be valid. The views expressed in this work are solely those
of the author and do not necessarily reflect the views of the publisher,
and the publisher hereby disclaims any responsibility for them.

Any people depicted in stock imagery provided by Getty Images are models,
and such images are being used for illustrative purposes only.
Certain stock imagery © Getty Images.

ISBN: 978-1-9736-8276-9 (sc)
ISBN: 978-1-9736-8275-2 (e)

Print information available on the last page.

WestBow Press rev. date: 5/8/2020

{My seriousness}

1. Even though my Health is changing, my Heart is still the same.

     I Love you.

2. *Do not let my diagnosis dictate our relationship.*

I Love you.

3. *Whispering makes me feel as if you have a secret that you cannot tell me. I used to help keep the secrets, now I feel like I am the secret.*

I Love you.

4. I remember when you used to look up to me, does it hurt you to look at me now?

I Love you.

5. I know it can be shocking to hear some of the words that come out of my mouth, believe me when I tell you, they're not coming out of my heart. I apologize in Advance.

I Love you.

6.   *Am I still your Hero?*

                        I Love you.

7.   *I need you to be tough for me, such as I have been tough for you. We are family and we're in this thing together.*

I Love you.

8. Remember all the good times that we used to have? Let's do it again...

I Love you.

9. *I am still who you need me to be in your life, even if I may forget who I am at times,*

I Love You.

10. *My world is not always BIG enough for the both of us. Sometimes, it's okay if I have my way.*

I Love You.

11. It is not my plan early in the morning, nor it
     is my goal in the midnight hours to cause you
     frustration.

     I Love You.

12. *Please continue to bear with me while WE fight this thing together.*

I Love You.

13. *FYI I don't hug with my arms I hug with my heart. When we Embrace, I'm giving you all of me. Embrace the moment.*

I love you.

14. *This is a good time to start singing some of my old favorite songs.*

I Love You.

15. *If I didn't like correction when I was a child,
chances are I'm not going to like correction right
now. PLEASE be patient with me.*

I Love You.

16. *Some of my views on life may change. Don't take it personal when I begin to embrace someone or something that you've never seen me embrace. I just want to love life again.*

I Love You.

17. *I know at times you wish you could have the old me back. If I could be honest sometimes, I wish I could have the old me back. Please don't let this scare you away from me.*

I love you

18. Be patient with your brother and sister. It's hard
	for them to see me like this. Just be patient.

I Love you.

19. *I may never tell you and if I do, you may not understand...BUT you are one of my Heroes and I thank you for all that you are doing for me.*

I Love you

{My Jovial Silliness}

20. Believe it or not, at times I still have a sense of humor. Some things I do on purpose just to make you smile. Hahaha

I Love You

21. How ironic, you used to keep me up all night
when you were a child. Now it's your turn to stay
up all night... BUT remember who's the child and
who's the Parent. Hahah

I Love You.

22. *Chances are, I will not tell you how horrible you sing at times. Hahaha*

I love you

23. *My steps are getting shorter but I will keep walking as far as you can lead me. Ps. And as far as I feel like walking because I'm still the Boss!!! Hahaha*

I Love You.

24. *Please do not panic when you see me coming cutie pie, because your face makes me nervous also!!! Hahaha*

I Love You.

25. There's a good chance I would like you to dress
me the way that I would like to dress myself. Just
consider yourself my personal assistant and
designer. Hahaha.

   I Love you.

26. I promise you do not bore me. I really am sleepy every time you come around. Hahaha.

I Love you.

27. *Watch your tone there little buckaroo, You too Missy. Haaaa*

I love the both of you.

28. *At my new place, my new friends keep better secrets than some of my old friends. Hahaha.*

I Love you.

29. *Don't be fooled. This fire is still burning. It's my way or the highway. Hahaha.*

I Love you.

30. *We are in this thing together, we are family, and I'm still part of your future! WHETHER YOU LIKE IT OR NOT HAHAHA*

I LOVE YOU.

31. *Are you asking me or telling me? HaHaHa*

I Love you.

32. *I'm sorry, but taking a shower is not quite like swimming regardless of what you think! Take your time with me in the water. Hahaha*

I Love you.

33. *Believe it or not, I might just start liking your cooking after all. Hahaha*

I Love you.

34. Confession: some things I am purposely forgetting. Haha have a blessed day.

I Love you.

35. *If you play some music, I might make it worth
    your wild. Hahaha*

I Love you

36. *Well it's not going to clean itself, so straighten your face up and get to it chop chop. Hahaha.*

I Love you.

*Please add Pic of Loved One during their
education or occupational days...*

37

Please add Pictures of your Loved one
Smiling & having a Good time

*Please add Pictures of you & Your Loved
One that Puts a Smile on your Face*

*Which of the 36 quotations registered most
with you & your Family? Why this quotation.*

If you and your Family could add a 37th quotation,
what would you add? (Serious or Jovial)

41

Last but NOT least important. Please write
a brief Love Letter to your Loved one.

Please all ow me to say Thank you to God, UT Health Science Center (Stakeholder Advisory Council), PCORI, Heart of Texas Hospice, and all the Many Families across this World that are trying to Keep it Together (We will keep it Two-Gether). To all those impacted by Dementia, just in case you did not know it, you still make a difference in your Loved One's Life.

Special Thank you to Mercer M. Butler (the late Retired Sgt. Brady M. Butler Sr.), NaShyra L, Josiah Emmanuel, & Ahmeir Taji.